Adrenal Fatigue

*Combat Adrenal Fatigue
Syndrome Naturally and Boost
Your Energy Levels for Good!
Reset Your Natural Balance Now!*

Jessica Forrest

Table of Contents

Introduction

When asked, most people do not know what adrenal glands even are, let alone what their purpose is and why they are important. Since many are not aware of these facts, they are also not aware of how to properly take care of their adrenal glands, and thus, how to properly take care of themselves.

When someone's adrenal glands are not working properly, it can cause problems. Our adrenal glands are extremely important and play a very big part in our overall wellbeing.

We have two of them, and they play a very big, very important role in producing some of the hormones that our bodies need. The times that they actually do the most work is during the times that our bodies are under stress.

The adrenal gland is most commonly known for its ability to produce and regulate sex hormones, as well as the "fight or flight" response. This is a physiological reaction. It only occurs because of a preserved threat, attack or harmful event. It is also sometimes called "the acute stress response".

It first began as a theory that animals will react to threats by a discharge that happens in the nervous system. As we well know, this takes place in humans also. All of the hormones that are secreted by one's adrenal gland will determine how they are able to respond to stress.

They are located right above your kidneys, in the middle of your lower back. Each person has one adrenal gland for each kidney, they are paired up, so to speak. Your adrenal glands actually influence your kidney function very strongly, due to the aldosterone that they secrete. The word "adrenal" stems from 'ad renes', which is Latin for "near the kidney."

One of the adrenal glands, the right one, is shaped like a triangle. The left adrenal gland is shaped more like a crescent. This is due to their vascular connections. The shape of each gland should not be a cause for concern, however, unless of course one or both are found to be enlarged.

They have a yellowish tint to them and they are roughly 1-inch-long and 2.5 inches wide. Each adrenal gland has three different parts, the capsule, the cortex and the medulla. The roles of the cortex and the medulla are very separate from one another; however, they do still interact with each other.

The adipose capsule is a layer of fat that surrounds the adrenal gland. The capsules primary responsibility is to protect the glands themselves and keep them safe. It works almost in the same way that an orange peel protects the orange fruit.

It is actually not technically part of the adrenal gland itself, its main function is to simply close it off and keep it safe from harm and any type of trauma or contamination. The cortex makes up about 80% of the adrenal gland. It completely surrounds the medulla, which is at the very center of the adrenal gland.

The cortex has three different roles. One role is to produce sex hormones and the hormones DHEA, DHEA-S as well as androstenedione. This takes place in the zona reticularis, which is the center part of the cortex. In men, these are the hormones that are later converted into testosterone. They are also in charge of the male hormones in women.

The zona fasciculate, the middle of the cortex, is responsible for our corticosteroid levels. This is extremely important because our Cortisol and all of its compounds are what control our sleep/waking cycle, regulate our blood pressure, generate energy from different foods, as well as work to suppress inflammation. People cannot live without these hormones.

The last section of the cortex, the zona glomerulosa, which is the outer layer, produces a hormone called aldosterone. This hormone regulates both our mineral and fluid excretion.

Although the medulla is small, making up only 20% of the entire adrenal gland, it is no less important than the other sections.

The function of the medulla is to manage our stress. The medulla produces three different hormones, referred to as catecholamines. These are epinephrine (most commonly known as adrenaline), norepinephrine, and dopamine.

These hormones are also known as neurotransmitters, or in some cases, "stress hormones." These are the hormones that create our basic stress response (which is part of our instincts) and helps keep people alive if and when they are being traumatized or they are in danger.

When a person is in a very stressful situation, their brain will immediately send a signal to their adrenal gland. The adrenal gland will then react by releasing stress hormones. This does a lot of different things. Some of them are increasing our awareness, diverting blood flow to our brain and muscles, and slowing down our digestion.

When the adrenal gland is not working properly, it can cause a lot of problems. It can produce too much of a hormone, too little of a hormone and/or cause the person to have several different disorders. One of the main disorders related to the adrenal gland that many people suffer from, is called "Adrenal Fatigue."

Adrenal Fatigue is the name given by doctors to describe fatigue and other symptoms that they believe are caused by an adrenal gland that is not working properly in people who are under stress, whether it be physical, mental or emotional. Many people say that this is actually not a proven medical condition since the main function of the adrenal glands is to produce hormones.

Chapter One

Adrenal Fatigue - What is it?

To put it very simply, Adrenal Fatigue Syndrome occurs when the adrenal glands are no longer able to cope with the amount of stress a person is under. It has existed just as long as we have.

However, it is much more common today. The reason for this can be explained through the drastic changes in our lifestyles. We used to sleep more, eat healthier, not consume nearly as much caffeine and sugar, our stress levels were lower and the amount of toxins around us was *significantly* lower.

There are four stages of adrenal fatigue. They are beginning the 'Alarm' phase, continuing the 'alarm' phase, the 'resistant' phase and the 'burnout' phase. During the first phase, the 'Alarm' phase, the body is reacting to an immediate threat.

This could be something as extreme as a hospital stay or a divorce, or even something as simple as an interview. The body makes very large amounts of hormones during this stage. If any labs were conducted during this phase, the results would show elevated levels of several different hormones, such as insulin, DHEA, cortisol, norepinephrine and adrenaline.

A person's body becomes much more aware and has an increase in arousal during this stage. It is very common that a person in this phase would not be able to sleep well. Usually, no one complains of any symptoms during this stage and many people will enter into this stage several times during their lives.

During the second stage, the continuing 'alarm' phase, the person's body continues to react to the stress that they are under. The endocrine system is still able to produce the hormones that the person needs but the levels of DHEA and sex hormones will begin to drop during this phase.

The adrenal gland uses the same resources to produce stress hormones as it does to produce sex hormones. Therefore, the levels of sex hormones begin to decrease because all of the adrenal glands resources are being put towards producing stress hormones.

It is during this stage that a person would begin to feel real effects of what they were going through. Many people being to develop an unhealthy addiction to coffee at this point. They will feel extremely wired but will be unable to calm down and go to sleep, regardless of how tired they may be.

During stage three, the 'resistance' phase, people will continue to have a drop in different hormone levels. At this point they would still be able to function as far as being able to keep a job and perform their normal daily activities.

However, they will begin to notice something really "just isn't right" with them. They will experience lack of enthusiasm, excessive tiredness, lower sex drive and even regular infections.

Many people will confuse this stage with depression, seeing as many of the symptoms are also symptoms of depression and it is very well recognized, while adrenal fatigue is not. This phase can unfortunately, sometimes last for years.

During stage four, also known as the 'burnout' phase, a person crashes after dealing with stress for such a long period of time. During this phase, an individual will suffer from weight loss, depression, anxiety, a disinterest in the world, apathy, irritability, lack of sex drive and extreme tiredness. At this point, the body will no longer be able to produce stress hormones. This means that sex hormones *and* stress hormones will drop significantly.

Symptoms
Since many doctors are not properly diagnosing their patients, many are being to be a lot more proactive. They are doing the appropriate research, documenting their symptoms and self-diagnosing.

There are many symptoms that are associated with adrenal fatigue. All of them will be listed, but the main concentration will be on the most common ones because there are so many of them.

Some of the most common symptoms of adrenal fatigue include:

- Difficulty getting up in the morning
- High levels of fatigue each day
- The inability to handle stress
- Higher energy at night
- Craving salty food
- A weak immune system.

Some of the other, less common symptoms are: allergies, respiratory complaints or asthma, dry skin, dizziness, dark circles under the eyes, joint pain, extreme tiredness after an hour long workout, frequent urination, lines in the fingertips, low blood sugar, low blood pressure, loss of muscle tone, lower back pain, low sex drive, weight gain, and numbness in the fingers or poor circulation.

Chapter Two

Why it's Hard to Get Help

Adrenal fatigue is still considered a controversial subject, due to the fact that many people do not consider it to be a real disorder. Although it is becoming more and more common, there are still a very good amount of doctors who are unwilling to give this diagnosis.

There are several different reasons for this. The first reason is that lab tests are very inconclusive. In order for the tests to come back with the correct information, a person's cortisol and DHEA levels would need to be tested several times throughout the day. This is because they both fluctuate so much during a 24-hour period.

The second reason this diagnosis is not more commonly given out is because most of the time, doctors are actually discouraged from giving it. They are discouraged both by commercial pressures, as well as insurance companies.

When it comes to insurance companies, every disease has its own code. They are known as the International Classification of Disease codes. They are given out by the World Health Organization. They do not yet have a code for Adrenal Fatigue, most likely because all of the labs that doctors have been giving to try to diagnose it come back inconclusive.

Chapter Three

Common Causes of Adrenal Fatigue

There are several major causes of Adrenal Fatigue. As you continue reading, you might realize that you have as many as two or three (or maybe even more) of these factors. However, please keep in mind, that since everyone's body is so different, some people can come down with Adrenal Fatigue from just one factor.

This does not come on suddenly. Adrenal Fatigue happens very gradually over time. In most cases, it takes *several years* before someone's adrenal glands become depleted. As you read through this list of causes, please take your past into consideration.

There could have been an event or a long term issue in your life that took place years ago that may have started your adrenal glands on this slippery slope.

Emotional stress is at the top of the list for causes for Adrenal Fatigue. The other major causes include insufficient sleep, pollutants and chemicals, chronic disease, trauma, and of course, diet. Let's explore each of these a little more closely.

Emotional stress is the number one cause for health problems, in general, especially Adrenal Fatigue. It can come from almost any source, relationships/breakups, work, your colic baby keeping you up at night, your teenager getting involved with the 'wrong crowd', the illness of a family member, you name it.

This is referred to as low-grade stress. People don't seek help with these issues because they feel as though they can manage them themselves. And they can, at least for a while. Low-grade stress can be managed short-term, but if it continues long term, the effects it has on your health can be horrible.

*There are many coping mechanisms to help someone deal with stress, which we will go over later in this book. However, the best way to deal with your stress is to eliminate what is causing it, if that is at all possible, and it usually is. Eliminating the cause of your stress might seem overwhelming or even impossible. It might seem scary, but more often than not, it can be done. You might need to change jobs, leave an unhealthy relationship, seek some professional help for your child, or it could be as simple as learning new organizational skills and putting strong boundaries in place. Take a few minutes to evaluate what is causing you stress and brainstorm some solutions for each one. Although making these changes might seem difficult, in the long run, it may also be the best thing for you. Your health, for one thing, will definitely thank you. *

The next cause for Adrenal Fatigue is insufficient sleep. Like stress, this affects most of us. The majority of Americans do not get nearly as much sleep every night as their bodies need to be healthy and function at the highest possible levels.

The first sign that your body is not getting enough sleep is when you are struggling to find balance between work and home life, and you just can't seem to get everything done, when you feel "there just aren't enough hours in the day."

Many of us try to stay up later and wake up earlier in order to do more and be more productive and effective. Actually, what we are doing is burning ourselves out. Due to lack of sleep, we get confused easier, become more irritable faster and are usually more sluggish during the day.

People often feel sick, getting headaches and feeling nauseous. They chalk it up to needing more coffee, and by drinking more coffee continue to make their bodies work harder and their situation work. The average American gets six hours of sleep per night, but if you are in the early stages of adrenal fatigue, it is very likely you are getting much less than that. Your body doesn't need coffee, it needs *rest*.

The human body has a fantastic ability to self-heal, if we will only give it the time it needs and allow it to do so. So, set regular work hours, cut out that late-evening movie, turn off your laptop and get some sleep!

Another cause of Adrenal Fatigue is pollutants and chemicals. The load of toxins that gets put into our bodies is astounding. Toxins are everywhere. There is antibiotics in the meat we are eating, pesticides are being sprayed on your vegetables, chlorine is put into the water we drink...there are even pollutants in the air!

It has been estimated that 2,000 chemicals are being introduced each year. Some of these are going into different products that we purchase, some of them are being put into our food, but did you know that only a very few amount of any of these chemicals are being tested for safety?

All of these chemicals are coming from different sources, but they are being mixed together in the human body. They are leading people to contract heart disease, cancer and even Alzheimer's. These chemicals affect the digestive system and immune system and are making people everywhere sick. A large number of these chemicals drastically alter the functioning ability of the adrenal glands.

Chronic disease is most definitely considered a long-term stressor to our adrenal glands. Any diseases that causes chronic pain cause the adrenal glands to become overworked. Even the illnesses that might seem less of an issue or easier to manage, such diabetes or asthma, will make your adrenal glands work harder and become exhausted much more quickly.

Trauma is usually not a long-term stressor. However, it does put a lot of extra stress on the body. Any kind of severe physical trauma can be very damaging and impact the body, even for years afterward. This does not have to be something as traumatic as a major car accident, it could surgery, or anything that causes physical harm to and puts stress on your body.

We will be reading about nutritional advice in the next chapter. However, since diet plays such a large part in a person's overall health, I would like to talk briefly about diet in this chapter, and how it may be causing your adrenal fatigue.

We've been told our whole lives "you are what you eat." We know how important the food we are putting into our bodies is. We know we need vitamins and minerals, fruits, vegetables, whole grains and proteins. Yet, the majority of people today are not getting what they need- nutrition. We eat more sugar now than we ever have before. We put it in everything, breads, cookies, cereals, oatmeal, what we drink, some people even add it into their spaghetti sauce!

In the 1800's, people consumed on average about 1-2 pounds of sugar a year. Today, on average, people consume around 150 pounds of sugar every year. The makeup of the human body has not changed during these last 200 years, but what we are eating sure has.

In order for our bodies to deal with the massive amount of sugar we are consuming, they are forced into producing more insulin and cortisol. Producing more of these hormones puts extra stress on both the adrenal glands and the pancreas.

Everyone knows that the more sugar you eat; the more weight you gain. Weight gain is also a contributing factor when it comes to Adrenal Fatigue. Usually, heavier people feel more tired and the ones who are more in shape feel more energized.

The fatigue associated with weight gain could very well also be a sign of Adrenal Fatigue. Extra weight puts more stress on your body and all of your organs, including the adrenal glands.

Chapter Four

Nutritional Advice for Combating Fatigue

There are two great things about the Adrenal Fatigue Diet Plan other than the fact that it will help you recover from adrenal fatigue. One is that it normally doesn't cost more than any other sort of diet.

The other is that it has numerous additional health benefits. There are two different aspects to this diet. The first aspect is that any foods that would make someone's Adrenal Fatigue worse need to be avoided.

The second aspect is that every food that aids in the recovery process should be sought out and should be actively eaten by the suffering individual. Meals should also be eaten around the same time every day. People should avoid any food to which they have an allergy or intolerance.

Whole foods should also be added to every meal, as much as possible. Some examples of whole foods are apples, peaches, grapes, bananas, mangos, figs, lemons, dandelion greens, kale, carrots, tomatoes, squash, eggplant and yams.

For people that suffer from Adrenal Fatigue, eating breakfast is extremely important. Usually, by the time someone sits down in the morning to eat breakfast, they have already been fasting for roughly twelve hours.

The human body needs fuel, it has to be the right kind and it also needs to last the entire morning. The patients' breakfast should consist of a mixture of high quality protein and a small portion of carbohydrates. Omelets make a fantastic breakfast for anyone with Adrenal Fatigue. The usual cereal and pancakes should definitely be avoided.

Many people with Adrenal Fatigue have low blood sugar. To help with this and avoid crashes, patients should try to eat several small meals all throughout the day. Since excess sugar is controlled by cortisol, eating anything with a lot of sugar should really be avoided.

Caffeine stimulates the adrenal glands to make them produce hormones in the very same way as during a "fight or flight" reaction. It puts a lot of stress on the body. Many people will get to the point where they feel as though coffee simply does not work for them. This is only because their adrenal glands are already so depleted that they cannot respond to the stimulus of the caffeine. It is very important to stop consuming caffeine if a patient really wants to recovery from Adrenal Fatigue fully.

Thankfully, the withdrawal symptoms usually only last about a week.

Fermented drinks are actually very good for digestive health and the immune system. Although they are not very popular in the United States. They can sometimes be found in health food stores. There are also recipes and step by step instructions that can be used to make them at home. They provide a lot of healthy bacteria to improve nutrient absorption and digestion. They are also very rich in minerals.

Even though seaweed is definitely not a staple food item in most homes across the United States, it is very rich in phytonutrients and minerals and believe it or not, most grocery stores sell it. Most people will normally not be able to get these from anything else they are eating. Patients should attempt to eat a wide variety so that they can try to get the most benefits possible.

By making bone broth, we can mimic the way our ancestors used to incorporate the bone marrow from animals into their diets. Back in the day, nothing went to waste. It provided nutrition that was considered extremely valuable and was often given to the sick. Research has shown just how important bone broth is.

It boosts the immune system, promotes healthy cholesterol and reduces inflammation. The amino acids, vitamins and minerals it contains are considered essential for good health.

Food sensitivities are important if you have Adrenal Fatigue. This is because the food sensitivities prevent the human body from both being able to absorb and use the nutrients it needs, while at the same time making the body's sleep/wake cycle harder to regulate and at times, even causing inflammation.

Food intolerances, allergies and sensitivities will also keep the gut from being able to digest and excrete food correctly. Since an intolerance, sensitivity or allergy will prevent a person's body from properly absorbing nutrients, it can leave the person in a weakened state, causing very low energy.

They can also cause the growth of unhealthy bacteria within the patient's gut which would continue to weaken their immune system even more. There are a few simple steps that an individual can take to deal with food intolerances and sensitivities. The patient can avoid that particular food, take supplements to aid in digestion and take supplements to strengthen the gut.

Adrenal Fatigue causes not only hormones deficiencies, but vitamin deficiencies as well. Although lab tests may show that someone who is suffering from Adrenal Fatigue is still within the normal range for various vitamins and minerals, people can tell a lot about how their bodies *feel*. If a person is continuously suffering from excessive tiredness and lack of energy, there is a good chance that they are suffering from a vitamin deficiency, or perhaps even multiple, caused by the Adrenal Fatigue.

Natural Remedies
There is a various amount of supplements, probiotics and herbs that can aid in the Adrenal Fatigue recovery process. The supplements that I would recommend are high-quality supplements.

There are many different brands of each vitamin on the market. They are not all the same when it comes to quality, safety and how well they work. Vitamins come in different forms, such as pills powders and liquids.

Which one you should take largely depends on how they work in your body and your personal preference. If you are unsure of which form you should take, your physician can explain to you the positives and negatives of each form and together you can decide which would be best for you.

They will also be able to tell you what brand are of the best quality. When the correct combination of high-quality supplements is used in partnership with the appropriate lifestyle and dietary changes, the journey towards reversing an Adrenal Fatigue condition becomes significantly smoother.

There are several vitamins that people with Adrenal Fatigue seem to lack. Some of them are vitamin B5, vitamin B6, vitamin B12, Vitamin C and magnesium. The B vitamins are very important in regards to cell metabolism.

If a person is able to boost their metabolism, it will, in turn, increase energy levels and reduce some of the fatigue that so often occurs during Adrenal Fatigue Syndrome. B% will work to create coenzyme A. This will directly contribute to the breakdown of fats, carbohydrates, proteins and assist in cellular respiration.

B6 contributes to the creation of adrenal hormones. B12 assists with cell repair, the maintenance of red blood cells and energy production. Since all of these B vitamins are different, the amount that a person would need of each one would also be different. There are some very good B-Complex vitamins that actually combine all three of these B vitamins that can be very helpful.

Vitamin C is an extremely powerful antioxidant. It is involved mainly in the production of cortisol. It has many other health benefits as well, such as protecting from free radicals and boosting the immune system. It is an essential building block when it comes to the recovery of the adrenal glands. Many people begin with 1,000mg of vitamin C per day and then begin to gradually increase.

Research has shown us that about 75% of all Americans are deficient in magnesium. Magnesium assists in maintaining energy flow. Therefore, a direct link can be seen in a magnesium deficiency and very low energy levels. Some of the other symptoms of a magnesium deficiency are depression, stiffness, muscle cramping and even insomnia. However, if someone takes too much magnesium, it can then cause digestive issues, so patients are advised to be careful when they are taking it and not to take more than is recommended.

It has been proven that probiotics are extremely good for our bodies. They can reduce side effects that may be brought on by antibiotics, improve our ability to digest food properly and they may even assist in lowering stress levels.

They are good for everyone, but they are most especially good for people with Adrenal Fatigue since they suffer from poor digestion. Probiotics are live bacteria (the healthy kind) and are directly linked to several different health benefits.

When probiotics improve a person's digestive system, they are then able to better absorb all of the essential nutrients within their food. This will then allow the person to be able to maintain their energy levels better, as well as produce the hormones that their body needs to function properly.

Probiotics also help to support the body's immune system, which would prevent any type of illness someone may come down with if their immune system was weakened, from further weakening the adrenal gland. A good probiotic will contain a minimum of five strains of bacteria, including Lactobacillus acidophilus.

It is said that some probiotics may have a calming effect on the human brain. Over the years, studies have been done on mice in an attempt to get more information on the benefits of probiotics.

As a result of these studies, scientists found that the good bacteria from the probiotics seemed to actually alter the moods of the mice. The mice had reduced reactions to anxiety and stress. They also had much lower levels of stress hormones than the mice that were only receiving the placebo.

Since the probiotics have other numerous health benefits, I recommend using them even if you do not see a difference in your mood or how you react to stress. You can find them naturally. Some foods that contain probiotics are yogurt, dark chocolate, pickles, sauerkraut, kefir, miso soup, microalgae, kimchi, tempeh, and Kampuchea tea. If you would rather, you can also take a probiotic in the form of a supplement; a good one is called FloraTrex.

In order to get the most benefit from the entire recovery process, herbal supplements should also be used. Herbs have been used for centuries, in many different cultures around the world.

Their most common use is for an increase in and ability to maintain energy levels, which is just what suffer of Adrenal Fatigue needs. There are several herbs that would be strongly beneficial. They are ashwagandha, rhodiola rosea, Siberian ginseng, licorice root, and maca root.

Ashwagandha is categorized as an adaptogenic herb. Adaptogenic herbs are considered to be one of the most important type of herbs for humans. They help to increase a sense of overall wellbeing, improve the immune system, and most importantly, help to build up a stronger resistance to long-term stress.

It works to regulate several different systems in our bodies. They fight against fatigue and stress, improve a person's sense of peace. It is very helpful because it also regulates cortisol. If a person's cortisol is too high, this herb will lower it and if it is too low, the herb will raise it.

Rhodiola rosea works like a magical herb. It has a variety of uses. It can help with poor circulation, muscle tension, fatigue and depression. When someone's circulation is improved, the adrenal gland can much more easily produce increase levels of cortisol when it is necessary.

Siberian ginseng increases mental awareness and improves stamina. It can also improve energy levels. However, patients should be careful that they do not consume too much of it because it can also cause an increase in blood pressure.

Licorice root can be very helpful as well, however, just like the Siberian ginseng, it can also raise blood pressure. Some of the benefits of this herb are the fact that it will stimulate hormone production, increase a person's endurance and assist in maintaining energy levels.

Since many people who have Adrenal Fatigue also have low blood pressure, the fact that licorice root and Siberian ginseng increase blood pressure is usually not a problem. However, if someone is suffering from high blood pressure, they should not take either of these herbs.

Maca root helps with cortisol regulation too. It also helps with blood sugar. It assists our cells in being able to draw in hormones more effectively. If a patient has low hormone levels due to the Adrenal Fatigue, this herb will help with that.

There are several other supplements you should consider that may be of some benefit to you. They are Omega-3, CoQ10, D-Ribose and Acetyl -L-Carnitine. Many people have the correct amount of Omega-6 in their bodies while at the same time, having an Omega-3 deficiency.

This imbalance has been known to cause increased inflammation. An increase in inflammation requires the adrenal gland to produce more cortisol. Omega-3 can help relieve your adrenal glands from some of their workload.

CoQ10 is produced by your body naturally and then later on turned into energy. This energy is used to grow and maintain your cells. Some people who are very in to fitness say that CoQ10 will increase their endurance and help them to recover faster after a good workout. You can take this as a supplement, or you can simply try adding more meats to your diet, such as sardines and beef.

D-Ribose is another good supplement to consider. It, like many others, also works to increase energy levels. It is able to increase your level of energy *without* putting any extra stress on your adrenal glands, which is exactly what you need. Many people who suffer from Adrenal Fatigue Syndrome have found this supplement to be extremely helpful.

Acetyl-L-Carnitine works to increase a person's energy levels by increasing their metabolism. It increases the creation of different neurotransmitters, ones that people usually are deficient in. it also helps to produce energy by moving all of our fatty acids into the mitochondria. This is important because the mitochondria are the part of the cell that takes nutrients and turns them into energy.

Chapter Five

The Adrenal Reset Diet

There is treatment for adrenal fatigue. However, it does take a lot of time, patience, persistence and in some cases a complete lifestyle change. If adrenal fatigue is not treated the person suffering will simply continue in stage four.

As you can imagine, they would not have a very good quality of life at all. In many cases the individual's immediate family members suffer as well, due to the fact that the individual is not always very easy to deal with or enjoyable to be around.

Normally, recovering will take anywhere between six and eighteen months, but each patient is different and there is a very wide range between individuals. The time frame for recovery from adrenal fatigue cannot be summed up into one simple answer because there are several different factors involved.

If an individual is still in one of the early stages of adrenal fatigue, they should be able to recover much faster than someone who has already progressed to stage three or four. Believe it or not, it is actually very common for people to go through level one and two of adrenal fatigue as a result of different stressors, multiple times throughout their lives.

It is extremely common and just about everyone goes through at least the first and second stages, perhaps progressing even further, they just may not know it is an actual syndrome with a name. Most people just say they are overwhelmed or burnt out and don't realize the magnitude all of this is really having on their health and their lives in general.

However, in many cases, they are able to recover naturally within just a few months after the stress has passed and been dealt with. That is usually the time when someone may enter into counseling for a short period of time, perhaps a few months, or even just a few weeks, to help them "get their lives together".

If they are only in the beginning stages of Adrenal Fatigue Syndrome, a few counseling sessions and some extra sleep, or maybe a vacation, could be all it takes to get them feeling like their old selves again.

The treatment will take much longer if the patient has reached stage three. It is at this stage that the body's entire endocrine system is becoming extremely overworked and fatigued. Several of the person's hormones have begun to drop now and the diurnal cortisol cycle has been interrupted.

At this point, in order to fully recover, the person would need to implement lifestyle changes, diet and use proper supplements. When patients are already at this level, it normally takes at least six months before they are able to recover from Adrenal Fatigue.

When people are in stage four, it should be expected that treatment will take a minimum of twelve months. This is because both the ability to produce stress hormones as well as sex hormones has dropped drastically.

In order to recover from this stage, people need to go through lifestyle changes, dietary changes, and the use of supplements. It sounds daunting but don't worry, these are all things that your body desperately needs and are craving. Things like more rest, less work, better nutrition, relaxing hobbies and regular exercise. When all of these things are put together, it will get you to feeling great in no time!

There is a diet known as the 'Adrenal Reset Diet.' This is not a diet made of nutritious food; it's more of a diet from work and technology. In my opinion, this is the most important aspect in a person's recovery from Adrenal Fatigue Syndrome.

Technology can be a very good thing and aid in our productivity quite a bit. However, if it is used excessively, it can cause several different health problems and get us way off track to where we are supposed to be. Some of the health problems it can cause are poor sleep patterns (or an inability to fall asleep quickly, stay asleep, or get a deep sleep in general), problems with your eyes, and bad posture. It can also have a negative impact on your social skills.

It has been proven through various studies that the over-use of technology directly impacts the amount of face-to-face social interaction we get. Lack of adequate social interaction, exercise (which is at an all-time low, due to people always wanting to 'surf the net' and be stagnant for long periods of time) and deep, restful sleep all play a part in depression, which is another symptom of Adrenal Fatigue.

One of the best ways to 'reset' your body is to limit the amount of time you spend watching television, playing computer games and video games, and surfing the net.

It is vitally important to your recovery for you to try to cut out technology at night as much as you can. Scientists have proven that the blue light that is given off from computer screens, Kindles, IPads, IPhones and television actually causes insomnia by altering a person's circadian rhythm.

The circadian rhythm is the 24-hour cycle that all living beings go through. It is what regulates the sleep/wake cycle. If you are starring at a computer screen or watching a movie right up until you go to lay down at night, it will take a very long time for you to fall asleep. The light (and noises, if you were watching a movie) stimulate your brain waves and cause you to stay awake longer.

There are several things that you can try to put into place to create your own Reset Diet Plan. Some simple things you can do are to turn off your computer, television, Kindle, etc. at least one hour before you go to bed.

Just like trying to eat your meals at the same time every day is important, being sure to get to bed around the same time every night, and wake up around the same time every morning, is also very important.

If you are able to stay on a schedule, it will help to regulate your body much faster. You should strive to get at least 9-10 hours of sleep per night. That sounds like a lot, but that is really the amount of rest your body needs, at least for now, to be able to recover fully.

You have been running on empty for so long, you need to give your body a lot of tender love and care to help it get back on track and function at optimum levels. Experts say that you should make sleep a priority for at least two weeks.

I strongly recommend this, as it will definitely jump-start your recovery process. I know I can feel a world of difference in my daily performance when I am able to sleep through the night, verses when I am up late or need to get up multiple times through the night.

In addition to not using any electronic devices so close to bedtime, try to avoid using them first thing in the morning as well. Computer and television screens have been shown to speed up brain waves, so they are not good for you first thing in the morning.

The noise from an alarm clock will do the same thing. It jolts you out of a sleep and into a state of alertness that does not normally happen if you awake on your own, without the use of an alarm clock. It is actually best to let your body wake up naturally if you can, although most people do not have the freedom to do this.

If you are not able to wake up naturally, due to your work schedule or other responsibilities, you will most likely need to be going to bed at a much earlier time. For people in the later stages of Adrenal Fatigue who are severely sleep deprived, it is actually recommended that they try to take a long weekend and just sleep and rest as much as they can.

This may not be possible for everyone, but if you have a couple vacation days that you have been holding on to, now might be the time to use one, or even a couple.

Doing your best to set regular work hours, and to leave your work *at* work, is important. You can bet that your health, and your family, will thank you for this. Set regular work hours and during those hours do your best to eliminate any and all distractions.

This means no chatting on the phone with your friends about this upcoming weekend or browsing on Facebook looking at funny pictures. Of course, be sure to take small breaks and let yourself breathe for a few minutes if you are feeling overwhelmed, but you would be surprised how much more work you would be able to get done if you really set your mind to it and just focused on working to the best of your ability during these hours.

Make a personal rule, at least for a couple of months while your body is resetting, that whatever work does not get done during these hours, simply does not get done that day. Make a point to work on these projects or loose ends at the beginning of your work hours the next day. Practicing good time management skills is important, as well as setting good boundaries with supervisors and co-workers, and will ensure you do not fall behind in your professional life.

Since Adrenal Fatigue is caused by different types of stress, physical, mental and emotional, that means that some types of workout programs can cause more harm than good. They can even keep you from losing weight.

If you have Adrenal Fatigue Syndrome, high-intensity exercise is not the type of exercise for you. It will make your Adrenal Fatigue worse because it will greatly increase your body's production of cortisol.

Although it might make you feel better in the moment, you will actually be making matters worse. You will most likely see that even though you are burning more calories, your body might actually be blocking fat loss due to the increase in cortisol. If you are not yet in the later stages of Adrenal Fatigue and you are trying to stick to a high-intensity workout program, you may find yourself entering into the later stages of this syndrome much sooner than you would otherwise.

For people who suffer from Adrenal Fatigue, light exercise is best. Any light exercise that you can get outside is ideal. The natural vitamin D is very beneficial. It will assist in regulating your circadian cycle and help you to have a much sounder sleep at night.

It also helps to ward off depression and regular light exercise has even been proven to naturally treat anxiety in a lot of cases. During my time studying Adrenal Fatigue I have found that people who often spend time walking along the beach have much lower stress levels and are sleeping much better at night than those who do not.

Being part of a community is also an important aspect of recovery. People are social beings. Face-to-face social interaction is a need everyone has, for some it is stronger than others, but nevertheless we all have the same basic need for companionship.

This is another part of the recovery process that also helps people who feel depressed and/or anxious. In most cases, when someone is feeling depressed and they spend a few hours with a good friend or a small group (and possibly eat some type of delicious food) they will notice a significant difference in how they feel. The same holds true for people who are feeling anxious.

Being able to verbally discuss the matter that is causing you anxiety to someone you trust and you know cares for you and has your best interest at heart, helps greatly. Actually, when someone is completely isolated from other people, it is considered to be one of the most traumatic experiences a person can go through.

Taking time to do something you enjoy and have fun is another aspect you should be incorporating into your Adrenal Fatigue Reset Diet Plan. What things do you greatly enjoy but never have the time to do?

By eliminating computer and TV time before bed, it will give you some extra free time to do something you love. It might be a light walk, reading a good book (but be sure it's a book with actual paper pages), or painting. Whatever it is, make sure you make the time to do it.

It would be good to try to do a fun, relaxing activity right before bed. It will help to lower your stress levels and promote a more satisfying sleep. Believe it or not, by sleeping better and lowering your stress levels, thus actually making yourself happier, you will be able to be much more productive during your work hours!

Chapter Six

Tips to Aid Your Recovery

Since we know different stressors can begin to set off Adrenal Fatigue for different people, anything from a simple job interview to a long hospital stay due to an illness, it is vitally important to try to live a life that is as stress free as possible.

This may seem impossible in today's world, especially considering the fact that the current cost of living is so high that in most families both parents need to hold down full time jobs while raising children, and that the average adult is only able to get about six hours of sleep every night.

However, it is possible to manage some of your stress and there are several things that each person can do to eliminate stress as much as possible. Some of these things include limiting caffeine, getting adequate exercise and taking regular breaks from work and/or projects they may be working on to allow their bodies time to rest and their minds time to relax and recoup.

There is a vast variety of activities that can be used to relieve stress. Spending time with friends and family, sitting and talking over a nutritious meal, going for a walk, and taking a hot shower or a bath are simple ones that can be done at home. However, if you are at work all day, it is very unlikely that you will be able to just stop what you are doing to do one or some of these activities.

If this is the case, simply closing your eyes and taking several deep breaths, inhaling through your nose, holding it for a few seconds, and exhaling slowly through your mouth will help you relax. If you are in an office or somewhere where you have a little bit of privacy, you can close your door and do some light aerobics, such as jogging in place for a few minutes or doing some quick jumping jacks.

Even taking a little walk down to the water cooler for a sip of water or to the staff lounge for a fresh cup of coffee can do wonders to clear your mind. Playing soft classical music and using a Zen sand garden or small river stones can be a great way to help reduce stress. These things would also add some life to your office and help other people to feel more at peace upon entering.

The best way to manage stress at work is by having strong boundaries. Set regular work hours and stick to them. If you are already bombarded with projects and your boss asks if you can take on another one, say no. if a coworker is slacking, let them slack. Don't let other people guilt or manipulate you into taking on their responsibilities. You have enough responsibilities already. Everyone deals with short-term stress at work but when it becomes long-term, it can be hurtful to your mind and body.

Dealing with too much stress for too long is what got you to this point, so keep that in mind and, for the time being, focus on yourself and your recovery. If you are continuously becoming stressed at work, it might be a good idea to start keeping a journal in your desk or locker.

You can keep track of what is causing you stress and over time you will probably find common factors. You can then use those findings and brainstorm different ways to eliminate these stressors one by one. You can also try talking privately with your supervisor.

Everyone can relate to the feeling of being completely burnt out and run down, because everyone experiences it from time to time. Just be honest. Explain that you will continue to do high-quality work and put your best foot forward, but in order for you to be able to keep doing that long term; you need to take some time for yourself.

You can't keep staying late at night or coming in early in the mornings. You can't keep taking on so many projects. Explain very politely and respectfully that you feel you are being stretched too thin, and they are not only likely to be sympathetic to your situation, they may even relate, want to learn more and possibly even join in and begin their own Adrenal Fatigue Reset Diet Plan.

Reading is a fantastic way to both relieve stress, and depending on what you are reading, educate yourself about something also. Many people of faith have found that keeping a small prayer book or slips of paper with verses or inspirational quotes in their pockets can be very helpful. If you are feeling stressed, overwhelmed, frustrated or depressed, simply take thirty to sixty seconds (or longer) to review some of them.

There are several tips that you can put into practice that will help you to be able to manage the stress from home life better also. Some of these are not projecting, sharing chores, family activities, eating dinner together and of course effective communication. People communicate in different ways.

This means that the ways everyone expresses and *receives* love are different too. Make sure you sit down and have a private discussion with each of your immediate family members asking them if they feel loved, assuring them they are loved and asking them what makes them feel the most loved.

Taking notes may be helpful if you have a bigger family. Don't be too embarrassed to also explain to each of your family members what makes *you* feel the most loved. Families almost always want to show love to one another, they just might not always know how to do it. Make this a discussion a priority, even if it seems uncomfortable, because it will most likely improve your relationship and your home life in general, significantly if you are able to effectively express love towards each other.

It is important to not project your outside stress and anger onto other people. It is not your family's fault if you are stressed out at work. They will be understanding and forgive you for this if it happens once and a while, but it definitely should not be a regular thing.

If you are having issues at work, you need to deal with those issues. Your family will start to resent you and not want to be around you if you are angry and stressed all the time. What is even worse is that your family members might think there is something wrong within their relationship with you if you become distant while at home due to your inability to cope with overly stressful work days.

So, do your family and yourself a favor, and keep your work life at work. Use your time out of work to enjoy your home life with the ones that love you and doing fun activities to help your mind and body relax.

Family activities Family activities do not have to be anything elaborate or expensive. You can do simple things such as going for walks, playing board games, having a picnic in the park or your backyard, even coloring. Anything that brings you together as a family and allows you to bond over the time you spend together and the experiences and feelings that you share with one another is perfect.

Try to evenly divide the household chores among everyone in the family who is capable of doing them. This will not only help to reduce your stress levels, but it will teach your children a strong sense of responsibility and to take pride in hard work and in their living space.

If they try to put up a fight, patiently remind them that you would really like to be able to spend more time with them, and that you feel it is very important to do so, but there are still all of these different household chores that need to be done. Explain that since each of them lives within that living space, each should help to keep it running smoothly, and that the sooner it gets done, the sooner everyone can do something fun together.

Dinner time is one of the most important times of the day for families. It is a time of coming together and of sharing. It is a time to put away the worries of the day and just simply be together. S, on the night's that you aren't rushing to church, a parent teacher conference, soccer, ballet or karate practice, be sure to take some time to sit around that big old kitchen table to eat, talk and laugh together.

In fact, while you're making these adjustments and putting your Adrenal Fatigue Reset Diet Plan into practice, maybe you should think about cutting out one or several of these extracurricular activities too. Believe it or not, adults aren't the only ones that can suffer from Adrenal Fatigue Syndrome. Children are just tiny people, after all.

As we already know, the mind and body are linked. Our physical wellbeing greatly impacted our mental wellbeing, and our mental wellbeing greatly impacts our physical wellbeing. Doctors usually do not talk about mind over matter during an office visit with a patient, but it is useful. Meditation and deep breathing can do wonders for anyone, especially people who are burnt out and dealing with stress.

Meditation is a practice. Meaning, you need to take the time to practice it on a regular basis in order for it to be effective. The person is working to train their mind so that they come to a realization of something, or for their mind to be able to recognize its own content without becoming fully wrapped up in that content.

Some use meditation to improve their focus, meditating for a certain amount of time and only allowing themselves to focus on that one subject of interest. Some people use different prayer beads while they are meditating, but this is not necessary. There are so many benefits of meditation that it is difficult to list them all.

A few of them are that it will lead to a much deeper level of physical relaxation, it reduces anxiety attacks, and it reduces virus activity and emotional stress, and improves the quality of the immune system.

I strongly recommend some kind (any kind that fits your personality and lifestyle the best) of meditation for everyone, whether they suffer from Adrenal Fatigue Syndrome or not. There are well over one hundred benefits to this practice and absolutely no negative side effects. It can be done in as little as ten to twenty minutes per day (longer if you would like, or shorter if you don't have a lot of time). It is not difficult to do because there is really no right or wrong way to do it.

There is a reoccurring theme throughout this book that a person's stress is directly related to an individual's health. Being able to effectively manage stress will help to not only recover more quickly from Adrenal Fatigue, but it can help to prevent it altogether.

Conclusion

The adrenal glands are a very important part of the human body. We rely on them for many different things and it is important to take care of them. All too often though, instead of taking good care of them, we actually take advantage of them. Taking care of them is not difficult to do.

The things that are needed to be done regularly in order to ensure they are functioning properly can just sometimes be a challenge for some people to put into daily practice. Once these things are put into place, however, it won't be long before these conscious decisions become second nature. Taking care of yourself is important. Take the time to do it.

www.ingramcontent.com/pod-product-compliance
Lightning Source LLC
Chambersburg PA
CBHW060650290526
45793CB00001B/480